BLISSFUL BATHTIMES
therapies for rejuvenating mind and body

Margó Valentine Lazzara

*The mission of Storey Publishing is to serve our customers
by publishing practical information that encourages personal independence
in harmony with the environment.*

Edited by Deborah Balmuth
Cover design by Wendy Palitz
Cover background illustrations by Alexandra Eckhardt
Cover image art © Juliette Borda
Text design and production by Susan Bernier

Table of Contents

Introduction

The bath is a special sanctuary from the troubles of our existence. It is a place to relax, to meditate, to let go of disturbing thoughts. Aromatherapy, combined with simple meditative exercises, can transform your bathing experience and increase your degree of pleasure.

This little book will show you how to create and use essential oil aromatherapy blends in the bath along with guided imagery, meditation, and visualization to stimulate and awaken the senses and to heal body, mind, and soul. Included are recipes for blends that — combined with specific practical exercises — will relieve stress, revitalize you, promote happiness and harmony, and increase your confidence. Allow the aromas to envelop your body, mind, and spirit.

Creating a Sacred Space

Ideally, your bathroom should be both a refuge from the turmoil and tensions of the outside world and a place of warmth and welcome. It should be a supportive environment in which you can accomplish your meditative aromatherapy baths in privacy and peace. First, clear out the clutter! Keep the room clean and fresh smelling. Throw damp towels that are hanging on the shower rod into the dryer and out of sight.

In creating your "sacred space," select and display objects of art, fragments from nature, or even candles — anything that will make the environment more inviting. Hang up inspiring pictures in unusual frames that will personalize your space, no matter how small your bathroom or budget.

For years I've collected interesting bottles, seashells, crystal bowls, trays for scented soaps, bath oils, salts, potpourri, and candles. I have an antique champagne glass in which I keep fresh lavender and tiny rosebuds, and I freshen the mixture with a few drops of lavender essential oil. Select objects with which you feel a connection. You can find exotic bottles at thrift shops and antique stores. You can purchase unscented bath salts and scent them with your favorite essential oil. The more attention paid to the bathroom, the more inviting it will become.

Bath Preparation

To make your bath the most beneficial and enjoyable experience possible, prepare in advance so that you don't have to rush around. Here are a few basic guidelines:

1. Wait a couple of hours after eating to take your bath. This will allow you time to digest and will facilitate your mind and body in achieving the full effect.

2. Rewrite each of the mental exercises found in this book on index cards in bold print or photocopy them for quick reference while in the bath. Cover the cards with clear tape or insert them into a plastic photo pocket so that they can be wiped dry for later use.

3. Have a nice fluffy towel ready for you after your bath.

4. Place a good no-slip rug by the tub to step onto upon exiting the bath.

5. Drink a glass of *room temperature* spring water before entering the bath and immediately after exiting.

Bring Nature Indoors

Plants and flowers enhance the beauty and tranquillity of your bathroom. Keep a small bunch of fresh flowers by the sink. Because I have a special emotional connection to gardenias, which were also my mother's favorite flowers, I like to keep a gardenia plant nearby. I also float gardenias in crystal bowls of water in the bathroom.

Select plants for their ability to thrive indoors, especially in the humidity of the bathroom. Avoid toxic plants if you have children or pets. Green and silver foliage is very relaxing, while reds and purples are more stimulating. It is also important to know the amount of natural light and temperature the plants require for their survival, so check with a nursery salesperson before choosing your plants.

Above all, make sure you will remain undisturbed for the duration of the bathing process. It is important that all activities be put on hold so you can devote your full attention to each mental exercise. This is not only quality time, it is also sacred time — time for you.

Entering and Emerging from the Bath

Be sure to add the selected oils *after* you have run a full warm bath, and then stir thoroughly to make sure the oil is evenly dispersed. Plan to remain in the bathtub for at least 20 minutes.

Light a candle of the correct color for your particular need (see pages 21–23). Do not step into the tub until the bath is fully drawn. Once the bath is prepared, remind yourself that it is your time to reaffirm your faith in yourself and your connection to your spiritual and emotional center. Use caution when entering and exiting the tub; sit on the edge of the tub and slide in. Slide down and, lying on your back, submerge the face, leaving the nose and mouth out of the water. You should stay in this position for as long as it takes you to complete the accompanying exercise.

Allow your body to relax in the scented water. Be sure to immerse your scalp to achieve the full benefits of the aromatherapeutic experience. Breathe in the aromas through your nose, hold your breath, then breathe out through your mouth. Take nice, long, deep breaths. Do this three times. Now you are ready to begin your visualization. Follow the guided imagery, meditation, or affirmation given with that particular bath. And enjoy the exquisite transformation!

When ready, emerge from the tub. Don't rush. Cover yourself in a soft towel; blot, don't rub, your skin. Alternatively, you could allow your skin to air dry.

The reaction to each bath is highly individualized, but the combination of the power of your mind and the power of essential oils can produce incredible results. You might emerge with more clarity and insight, a sense of deep relaxation, or a feeling of profound peace. Always block out time to be alone and introspective after a healing bath.

Bath Tips

Essential oil baths have a cleansing action that elicits a physical, emotional, mental, and spiritual response. It might take a little time before you see significant results, but the more you practice, the more you allow a deeper connection with your inner persona to develop.

The best time of day for a bath is when you know you won't be interrupted or distracted. The fewer distractions, the better your concentration. Keep the bathroom warm; your body temperature decreases while you are meditating. Turn up the heat or shut the windows; you will distract yourself if you have to run hot water during the bath.

Try to space baths at least two days apart if you are working with different moods. You can do the same bath every day for 7 to 10 days. Light a candle or dim the lights for ambience, but *do not fall asleep!*

 What If I Don't Like Baths?

If you prefer showers, you can still enjoy the healing effects of an aromatherapy blend. Make the bath blend in advance and put it in a plastic spray bottle filled with 4 ounces of distilled or spring water. After showering, spray yourself with the blend, avoiding the genital area, and let your skin air dry. Lying in bed in a quiet room, practice the deep breathing that is suggested for the bath, and then follow with the accompanying meditation and visualization.

Enhancing Your Life
with Aromatherapy

The bath became seductive and irresistible to me once I started using the different oils and beautiful extracts. You'll want to take a healing bath every day once you start adding these fragrant essential oils to your bathwater!

Essential oils give herbs, spices, fruits, and flowers their specific scents, aromas, and flavors. Each oil has individual benefits to which the mind, the body, and the spirit respond. Almost everybody benefits from the use of essential oils. Pure plant oils can improve your state of mind and generally enhance the quality of your life. What makes them beneficial is that they work in harmony with the body. Each oil has the ability to evoke different memories that can affect a person's physical, emotional, and psychological levels. Best of all, using essential oils boosts the immune system by combating the stress that ultimately weakens the body's resistance and makes you susceptible to illness.

Scents can trigger memories because of their quick access to the limbic system in the brain. It is here that scents will evoke an emotional response, such as hunger or sexual appetite. They can help you recall long- and short-term memories. If a particular scent stirs up past hurts or painful emotions and memories and causes you suffering, then you might want to avoid this specific scent. But I believe that it is good to be able to release this kind of hurt and pain rather than avoid it. Think about the scents that can bring about recollection of your past experiences.

How to Purchase and Store Oils

Essential oils are extremely precious and should be treated with respect. They also vary in cost depending on the plant; I have purposely eliminated jasmine and rose from the recipe bath blends because they can be very costly. While the lavender plant produces lots of oil, rose and jasmine produce very small amounts, and that affects the price.

When you have chosen the bath you would like, purchase the essential oils listed for it. Make sure the oils come in brown or blue glass bottles; the coloring protects them from decomposition caused by ultraviolet light. Purchase the smallest bottles in order to keep your expenses down until you discover your favorite bath blend combinations.

The experienced aromatherapist can tell just by smelling the oil whether it is high-quality or has been diluted with a carrier oil — such as jojoba, grapeseed, or apricot — so it can be used in a massage or perfume blend. Quality depends also on the method of processing and extraction: how and where the plant was grown and whether the right amount of pressure and steam was used during distillation. Just keep in mind that essential oils do vary tremendously, but you will still reap the benefits.

You might find oils or products that are labeled ESSENCE. These are chemically synthesized. You *do not* want these; although they might smell nice, they do not have the medicinal properties necessary for the baths described in this book. You should purchase only products marked PURE ESSENTIAL OILS and check the origin of the brand. Inhale some essential oils sold in health-food stores and pharmacies and buy those that appeal to you. Let your nose guide you.

Keep the essential oil bottles in a cool, dark place. This will prolong their shelf life. The optimum shelf life of an essential oil is about one year.

Blending Oils

When I embark on the adventure of making even the simplest blend, I eagerly anticipate the final product. Start with a cleared-off space such as a kitchen counter or table. Cover the area where you will place the open bottles of essential oil; any spillage can damage the surface of your table.

Most essential oil bottles have little plastic covers that allow only a drop at a time to come out, but if this is not the case, you can purchase eyedroppers for this purpose. Keep your different oil droppers separate; if you use a dropper for one oil and then use it for another, it can alter the blend. Instead, clean reusable droppers with rubbing alcohol and let them dry thoroughly. You also can soak them in vodka.

Most health-food stores carry "treatment bottles" for Bach flower remedies. These are empty, amber-colored glass bottles with their own eyedroppers. A box of four costs only $1.50. I find these most appropriate and affordable, and excellent for storage. A blend will keep for about three to six months if it is stored in an amber-colored bottle in a cool place away from sunlight. Storing for a longer period can cause deterioration of the rubber bulb on the dropper.

Once you've put the recommended amounts in the bottle and closed the cap tightly, swish the bottle around to blend the oils very gently, rather than in a vigorous manner. Remember: Essential oils are precious substances and energies that should be appreciated. Treat your blend as if it were liquid gold.

Cautions on the Use of Essential Oils

The oils I have recommended in this book have been carefully selected for their gentle healing properties. Adhere to my dosage instructions! Discontinue use if any irritation arises. When you are working with different essential oils, try not to expose yourself to too many of them at once for a prolonged period. I have found myself "scent-sory" overloaded from working with too many fragrances. Your body will tell you if you are overdoing it; you might get a headache or feel a little nauseous.

Pure essential oil can irritate or burn the skin, so use caution in handling and always dilute with a pure carrier oil — such as jojoba, apricot, safflower, canola, grapeseed, or olive — before applying directly to the skin. Be very careful not to rub your eyes after handling oil. Note, also, that any spillage on clothing will stain like perfume or other oil-based products. And always keep essential oils out of the reach of children. Do not use the bath blends if you are pregnant unless recommended by a qualified health practioner. Some oils may irritate the respiratory tract, so use caution if you have asthma or other lung conditions.

Enhancing Your
Bath Experience

Even today, the ancient Indian system of solar-ray healing still recommends therapeutic color baths. To make your own therapeutic color bath, purchase a colored lightbulb in the shade you need to evoke a particular mood. Avoid fluorescent lights; they emit pulsing flickers that can make you ill. Insert the colored bulb into your bathroom fixture or portable lamp and light it for use during your bath. Of course, if you are using a portable lamp, be sure it is a safe distance from water.

I like to use natural food coloring in my bathwater. Several drops added to the bath won't affect your skin and will tint the water to a gentle hue. A handful of fresh flowers provides you with a color energy bath. Let the blossoms float around on the surface of the water so they can visually stimulate you, rather than tying them up in a bag.

Candles are many people's favorite bath accessory. They are soothing and beautiful, and the flickering candlelight can bring a sense of peace and serenity to the room. Choose candles in colors that promote the mood you desire — turn the page for descriptions of each color's specific qualities and properties.

Specific Color Details

Each color has its own frequency and wavelength. The longest wavelength and the shortest frequency belong to red, and magenta has the shortest wavelength and the highest frequency. When you work with color, your body becomes sensitive to it and grows more open to meditation and healing. Color affects you physically, psychologically, and emotionally. In order for you to appreciate the power of color, you must know each color's particular attributes.

Red increases vitality and energy. This color is traditionally considered the seat of life-force energy; it is invigorating, vital, and activating.

Orange is cheerful, working as an antidepressant and creating a happy environment. Use orange when you need to facilitate the process of letting go. Orange can relax mind and body and loosen areas of stress.

Yellow has a detaching quality, creating a lack of involvement. It is uplifting, but a large amount of the hue induces nervousness and tension and can be disorienting or perplexing. Yellow has been known to distort perspective.

Green can cause hyperactivity without scattering your energy. It promotes sound judgment, stability, and physical equilibrium.

Turquoise is soothing, inviting interest and easing tension. This color helps release anxiety while providing support. Turquoise is refreshing and stimulating.

Blue is a relaxing color. It invites communication, meditation, and balance by calming the body and mind. Because blue creates softness, it is best used in stress-related areas such as the office.

Violet promotes self-confidence and love and concern for others. Use violet in meditation and prayer, or whenever you need to concentrate. It is the center of self-respect and pride and expresses individuality. Inner balance, silence, and relaxation are all aided by violet. A mind-balancing color, it helps you unburden and protect yourself. But violet is also an aphrodisiac and is widely used to promote festivity.

Magenta helps to raise energy levels. This color is impervious and forceful and is used to stimulate and inspire. Magenta brings self-respect, dignity, and composure by aiding and promoting concentration. It is also the color of spiritual love.

Visualization

Visualization starts in the imagination, where you form a mental picture of exactly what you desire to create in the universe. The more clearly you form the mental picture in your mind, the more accurately it will be produced as a physical fact. Using the techniques of visualization, you can restore yourself by building strong pictures of the healing taking place and the outcome that you seek. Work on strongly believing that these mind pictures are real.

By tapping into and using your thoughts in a more conscious way, you use your imagination to create and attract what your heart desires. You can have more loving and satisfying relationships, more rewarding work, more enthusiasm and enjoyment of every day. Stress reduction, increased health, wealth, a love of life, a love for other people, and a heightened appreciation for each and every day of your life can be attained — if you believe in yourself and want to accomplish it!

Simple Visualization Exercise

1. Select a pleasant warm room that is free of distractions. Lie or sit on a comfortable piece of furniture, a large pillow, or the carpet. You are now ready to take a mental "vacation."

2. Focus on the sound of your breath moving in and out. Feel the breath as it enters and then exits your body. Do this for about 1 minute.

3. Visualize yourself on an isolated mountaintop, looking out over the peaceful countryside. There is a cool, shaded stream running below. If you'd rather visualize another quiet spot that is special to you, do so. See, feel, smell, and taste your surroundings; linger on and enjoy every detail. Stay there for a couple of minutes, taking in the entire experience. Try not to let your mind wander from the scene.

4. When you are ready, bring yourself back to the room. You will be amazed at how much more relaxed and refreshed you feel.

Stress Relief
Bath

The more you know about stress, the better equipped you will be to minimize stress-related problems. Stress can ruin your day, and doctors are discovering that it can also ruin your health. When we are faced with a stressful situation, impulses sent to the brain via the nervous system activate the pituitary gland to secrete hormones into the bloodstream. These hormones activate the adrenal glands to secrete adrenaline and noradrenaline. This increases your blood sugar. Research has proved that when your tissues are soaked in stress hormones, your blood pressure, blood sugar, and heart rate skyrocket, while your capability for digestion and absorption shuts down.

Chronic stress increases your risk of everything from glaucoma to heart disease, and it makes you 50 percent more likely to catch the latest virus going around. Studies have shown that at least 80 percent of doctor's visits are for health problems that have been triggered by stress!

Stress Relief Blend

Soak away anxiety and stress — just add this blend to your bath. The most relaxing baths are warm, not hot! Hot water shocks the system, causing muscles to contract. Warm water calms you by increasing circulation and relaxing the muscles. Do not use this bath if you are asthmatic or pregnant — but do perform the accompanying visualization.

  3 drops bergamot essential oil
  2 drops clary sage essential oil
  2 drops lavender essential oil
  2 drops neroli essential oil
  2 drops sandalwood essential oil

Visualization Exercise: Stress Relief

✳ Run a warm bath and add the Stress Relief Blend; mix well. While you are in the bath, close your eyes and simply take a deep breath, being aware of the exquisite natural extracts you are breathing in. Breathe in calmness and exhale tension. Breathe with your belly, imagining that your lungs are sitting right behind your belly button. To fill them with air, relax your abdomen and let it expand with each breath. Slowly inhale for a count of 8, filling your belly, and slowly exhale to the count of 8.

✳ Do a few repetitions of this and then, starting with the top of the head, release the tension from your muscles one by one, all the way to your toes and back up again. Continue to breathe in relaxation and exhale tension.

✳ Now that your body feels soft and relaxed, allow your awareness to come inside yourself. Visualize yourself walking on a path among trees. In front of you is a gate. Open the gate and step into a beautiful garden.

* You see and smell beautiful flowers. You see lush palm trees, fruit trees, and tropical blossoms with sweet fragrances. Touch them . . . inhale the aromas. Each time you inhale, you feel more calm and relaxed. Listen to the singing birds. Feel the calm, gentle breeze.

* A wonderful feeling of peace and joy drifts through your mind and flows through your body. Visualize a magnificent cool waterfall. As you step into it, feel the clean, refreshing water cleansing you from the top of your head down to your toes, washing away every bit of stress and anxiety. Allow your being to be restored on all levels.

* Now project your thoughts forward. In a vision, see yourself in what might be a stressful situation, but allow the exquisite feeling of relaxation to continue to soothe your thoughts. Allow the relaxed state you are feeling now to weave a tapestry of a totally stress-free consciousness into your vision. Your mind and body are being conditioned to respond calmly to stress.

❋ Open your eyes slowly and exit the bath, taking with you this calm and relaxing feeling, and remembering you can always return to this peaceful garden of serenity that is your own private sanctuary.

Tips for Reducing Stress

Laughter is indeed good medicine. When you laugh, you actually cause a pleasurable change in your body's chemistry that lasts as long as 45 minutes. So take in a comedy at the movies, watch a funny television show, or invite friends over for a game of charades!

Pets can provide excellent stress therapy. The presence of pets and physical contact with them has proved to be therapeutic for hospital patients. Play with your dog, hold your cat, or sing to your bird; all of these activities can help reduce blood pressure and bring a feeling of calm.

The soothing, stress-relieving power of nature has been recognized for centuries. Many hospitals and health centers now make "nature areas" a part of their therapeutic environment. And when properly tailored to the individual's conditioning and enjoyment, physical exercise can help reduce stress and anxiety. Take a walk outside, or try hiking, biking, or rowing.

"Music hath charms to soothe a savage breast," wrote William Congreve back in 1697. Music's calming effect has been proved during dental procedures, during labor, before and after surgery, and in emergency rooms. This effect is probably due to music's ability to distract and soothe. Similarly, while daydreaming is often criticized, it can provide a refreshing break from tension. It can be as simple as recalling pleasant memories or envisioning an upcoming vacation.

Revitalization
Bath

One of the secrets to a long life is to continue growing, reaching, and changing. If you are physically weak, start exercising your body. Jog, hike, swim, play tennis — do whatever activities you enjoy that will give your body the movement it needs. You can reap enormous benefits from even a small amount of physical activity every day. Dancing is one of the best workouts and is an excellent tonic for your spirits, too. It enables you to freely and joyfully let go of physical and mental tension. Setting aside times for daily relaxation is a good investment. It results in renewed energy and vigor.

If your thoughts are weak, start exercising your mind. Meditation and guided imagery are healthful and natural foods for your mind. Practice these regularly to strengthen your concentration and ability to deal with stress. Your mind is the key to healing, regeneration, and a healthy glow.

If you desire a robust, energized, strong, healthy body, then think health and you will bring health. Nourish your mind as you nourish your body.

Revitalization Blend

To wake up in the morning or to refresh yourself after a hard day's work or before an evening out, this bath gives vitality to the physical body. If you are pregnant or asthmatic, do not use the bath — but do perform the accompanying visualization.

3 drops rosemary essential oil
2 drops bergamot essential oil
2 drops peppermint essential oil
2 drops thyme essential oil

Visualization Exercise: Revitalization

✳ Light a yellow candle; place it where you can see it, but not near anything that could ignite. Run a warm bath and add the Revitalization Blend; mix well. Climb in.

* Once in the bath, picture in your mind how blood circulates through the body. When it mixes with fresh oxygen, the blood is a vibrant, rich red color, but as it travels farther from the lungs, it loses oxygen and turns a dark shade of purple.

* Take a deep breath now and imagine that you are drawing in a massive amount of oxygen. As you exhale, you are blowing out useless carbon dioxide. Another deep breath invigorates the blood and draws oxygen deeper and deeper into fatigued tissues. Take another breath, stretch, and see the oxygen reviving and replenishing all the blood cells in every fiber of your body. Breathe in again and see your body saturated with oxygen: vibrant, alive, and refreshed.

* The golden yellow glow from the candle can nourish your soul, helping you regain your personal power and find your inner radiance. Envision this golden yellow as a bright sun sending you energizing rays, enveloping you. Feel it

restore and renew you inside and out. Remain in the tub for at least 15 minutes. Emerge from the tub when ready and extinguish the candle.

Tips to Keep You Feeling Revitalized

Get sufficient rest and sleep, and set aside time to practice deep relaxation.

Take a 5-minute "soother" — relax in an armchair and breathe deeply — before engaging in stressful activities.

Do as little as 20 minutes of aerobic exercise several times each week. Aerobic exercise allows endorphins — which have been called "the brain's narcotic" — to be released into the system. Endorphins let your mind soar free and keep you feeling good for up to 5 hours after exercise.

Happiness and
Harmony Bath

When do you feel most alive? Is it when you fall in love? When you see a sunset? When you listen to your favorite music? I want you to visualize a special moment in your life that brought you happiness and joy. Close your eyes and take a few minutes. Open your eyes. You can feel that feeling more often than you realize.

Give yourself permission to feel happiness without fear. However life is unfolding for you right now, there is within you some unknown source — a level of peacefulness with joy — that is beginning to express and expand itself. Experience the shift you feel when you change your perspective. You can access an enormous source of power.

Happiness is a condition of thinking as well, but being in the moment is an experience that you should permit yourself to have more of. Look forward to these times daily, hour to hour, moment to moment. Happiness and harmony are achieved in the way you respond to each and every day without focusing on the frustrations in your life. Change your perception when problems arise.

Happiness and Harmony Blend

This blend is good when your spirits are low and you are feeling depressed. If you are pregnant or asthmatic, skip the bath and proceed to the visualization.

- 3 drops bergamot essential oil
- 3 drops ylang ylang essential oil
- 2 drops clary sage essential oil
- 2 drops neroli essential oil

Visualization Exercise: Happiness and Harmony

✳ Light a pink candle (at a safe distance from flammable objects) or place a pink lightbulb in the bathroom fixture. Disperse the Happiness and Harmony Blend in the bathwater and mix well.

✳ Once you are immersed in the bath, inhale the sweet, refreshing, fruity aromas of bergamot, ylang ylang, neroli, and clary sage. Do some deep breathing until you feel your body relax.

✳ In this visualization, you will use the color pink. This color is uplifting and relaxing and should be used to encourage love and nurturing. Pink light is especially useful when you are feeling sad and lonely, unloved, depressed, or rejected, or when you are grieving. It provides much healing and nurturing of the spirit and the emotions, and it connects you with universal love vibrations.

* Gaze at the pink candle without blinking, and when you can no longer hold your eyes open, allow them to close, bringing that pink color into your inner vision. Place your hands over your heart and allow the color to permeate your heart and chest area. See yourself receiving what would make you happy and harmonious within yourself. See yourself giving and receiving unconditional love.

* Concentrate, focus, and visualize strongly. Visualize the pink flame burning vividly in your heart and repeat inwardly, then outwardly, the following affirmation: "I will be happy and harmonious under any and every circumstance. I am love. I am joy. I am forgiveness."

* Emerge from the bathtub when you're ready and extinguish the candle. After your bath, pull on a pink T-shirt, nightgown, pajamas, or nightshirt, or sleep on a bed dressed with pink sheets and pillowcases. The following day, wear the same color close to your body — a pink shirt or blouse is perfect.

Tips for Encouraging Happiness and Harmony

Stretch out and increase alertness before getting up. Start stretching your body while sitting on the edge of the bed. Roll your head in a circular motion, allowing it to fall forward, to the side, and back. Stand up with your arms toward the ceiling, fingers outstretched, and reach first on one side, then the other. Now hang your head and arms loosely toward the floor and allow gravity to pull you down slowly. Stretch your spine while trying to touch your toes, and hang in that position for a while.

At night, create a peaceful, soothing, relaxing atmosphere in your bedroom by lighting candles and spritzing essential oils throughout the room. Take care to extinguish all your candles before going to sleep.

Take time for breakfast. Breakfast is a source of energy, and you need it to replenish blood glucose levels in the brain.

Get sufficient rest and sleep. Eat well-balanced meals, and get regular exercise.

Visualize a positive and creative day ahead of you, and think of all the good things you have in your life. Look forward to the good things that are coming your way.

When people you love are pulling you in two directions, take a "time out" for yourself. Sitting quietly, tune out everyone else and follow your heart.

Flower Healing
Bath

Chakra is a Sanskrit word that means "wheel." The chakras are spinning vortexes of energy, the network through which body, mind, and spirit interact as a holistic system. By activating the seven chakras, you will release physical, mental, and spiritual blocks.

Energy created from our emotions and mental attitudes runs through the chakras and is distributed to our cells, tissues, and organs. By sending breath to the seven main chakra points, you open and charge each chakra and the surrounding organs with a vital life force. You direct breath to a chakra by focusing on the location of the chakra and visualizing the breath being sent to that area.

Chakras are doorways for our consciousness through which emotional, mental, and spiritual forces flow into physical expression. Each of the chakras is ascribed a dominant color and has a special link with one of the endocrine glands and a physical organ. The colors are the seven colors of the rainbow spectrum. Each assigned color, when visualized with focused breathing, activates the energy in the chakra.

Flower Healing Blend

Flower healing is the most powerful way to open, activate, energize, and balance all of our chakras. Do not use the bath if you are pregnant or asthmatic, but perform the accompanying visualization.

- 3 drops patchouli essential oil
- 3 drops ylang ylang essential oil
- 2 drops myrrh essential oil
- 2 drops sandalwood essential oil
- 1 drop peppermint essential oil

Use the Flower Healing Blend in conjunction with the following visualization to consciously expand your experience of unconditional love, gratitude, compassion, forgiveness,

The Seven Chakras

Chakra	Location	Color	Purpose
First (root)	Base of spine	Red	Aids in your survival and how you interrelate with the world.
Second (navel)	Just below belly button	Orange	Expresses feeling of vitality and increases sex drive and creativity.
Third (solar plexus)	Above navel (below rib cage)	Yellow	Vitalizes the nervous system and gives self-assurance.
Fourth (heart)	Center of chest	Green	Energizes the blood circulation. When this energy center is open, you feel compassion.
Fifth (throat)	Throat area	Blue	Facilitates communication.
Sixth (brow)	Center of forehead	Indigo	Increases intuition and insight.
Seventh (crown)	Top of head	Violet	Vitalizes the upper brain. You will feel a wonderful, joyous connection to everything and everyone around you. You will achieve great clarity and insight.

and creativity. During this meditation, you will visualize a particular color corresponding to each chakra to balance that part of your body. You will bring yourself more harmony, creating a sense of wholeness within yourself.

Visualization Exercise: Flower Healing

* Prepare a bath with the Flower Healing Blend, mix well, and light a white candle (near the tub, but safely out of reach of flammable materials). Accept its calming effects and spiritual qualities. Pull some white carnations from the stems and place them in the tub. Immerse yourself in the bath and breathe deeply. Allow your eyes to close; take a deep breath and hold it for a few moments. Release and repeat. Imagine the white flowers that are floating around you.

* Focus on the root chakra near the base of your spine. Imagine the color red as a spinning globe. Send your breath to the base of your spine and see it spinning, then opening up into a red flower. See the petals fluttering open. Focus on

the area just below your navel, your second chakra. Visualize a spinning ball of orange opening up into a bright orange flower, and see the petals fluttering and opening.

* Bring your attention up to your third chakra, above the navel. See a yellow, sunlike ball shining and spinning brightly, then imagine it opening up, petal by petal, into the brightest yellow flower. Concentrate on the center of your chest, the fourth chakra. See a ball of green glowing and spinning. When it stops, the green leaves open slowly.

* Focus on your fifth chakra, at the throat. Visualize a globe of sky blue that comes into your throat, spinning and becoming the loveliest flower. Watch as it opens up, petal by petal. Now concentrate on the "third eye" area between your brows. A spinning ball of indigo vibrantly glows and opens. Now all your attention should focus on the crown chakra at the top of your head. Visualize the color violet spinning and opening, releasing any pressure at the top of the head.

✳ Now see all of the brilliant colors spinning. A white pure light of energy cleanses you from the bottom of your spine through all the colors and out through the top of your head, and it cascades down to your feet. You are cleansed and balanced! Your consciousness will come to full awareness now.

Tips for Maintaining Balance

Eat fresh fruits and vegetables of the colors corresponding to the chakras.

Fast for short periods (1 to 2 days); do this *only* under the supervision of a holistic doctor.

Try the Flower Healing Visualization while standing, placing your hands over each chakra point and bringing sound to each rapid breath while visualizing the assigned color. This helps clear emotional blocks.

Increased Confidence
Bath

Lack of confidence can come from negative programming that has adversely affected your development. Perhaps a parent put you down, or a teacher failed to recognize your assets and potential, or a demanding employer fired you. Or maybe some of your own actions are responsible. You need to leave the past behind and not allow it to hold you back.

While you cannot make the events of the past disappear, you can change the perspective from which you view them — focusing on the positives instead of the negatives — to enable you to develop into the person you want to be. What you have accepted as failures were really learning experiences. Learning is essential to personal growth.

You can transform "nervous energy" into positive energy that you can consciously direct in a constructive way. For example, if you're nervous about giving a presentation, recognize that you can use that energy productively. Begin focusing your mind either by meditating or writing down a detailed plan of action. Do some deep breathing to slow down. Understand that your nervous feelings can be transformed into good humor, an entertaining speech, or a mental quickness that will help you answer questions. Channel that energy productively instead of scattering it all over the place and getting nowhere.

Increased Confidence Blend

Increase your inner strength with this blend. You will become more confident! If you are pregnant or asthmatic, skip the bath and proceed to the following visualization.

- 3 drops clary sage essential oil
- 3 drops myrrh essential oil
- 2 drops marjoram essential oil
- 2 drops ylang ylang essential oil

Visualization Exercise: Increased Confidence

* Draw a warm bath and add the Increased Confidence Blend; mix well. Light a blue candle (be sure the candle is not near anything that could catch fire) and climb into the tub. Breathe deeply and allow all your muscles to relax. Breathe deeply and take in the scents. With your eyes closed, visualize the color blue. Take another breath and allow your mind to daydream.

* You are at a gathering of people, conversing. Visualize yourself relaxed and composed, speaking and acting with self-assurance, secure in your own knowledge. Now see and hear yourself saying, "I'm confident! I'm successful! I'm goal-oriented! I'm a winner!" Vividly picture yourself confident and full of inner strength. Focus all your thoughts on this image for as long as you can.

* Now see yourself take new pride and joy in your growth and success with clear goals. For example, visualize yourself taking that night class that can give you the freedom to move forward. Or asking for that raise you deserve. Maybe you can see yourself making that public presentation you fear more than anything and actually becoming excited about the opportunity.

* Accept this suggestion deep into your subconscious mind, retaining it and believing it. By having allowed yourself to go into deep relaxation, focusing steadily and visualizing every detail of the desired outcome, you will bring it to fruition. Bring your awareness back to the present when you're ready.

Tips for Increasing Your Confidence

Use your imagination as a positive force. Imagine only positive outcomes.

Visualize only scenes of success in your mind and look on the bright side. You have nothing to lose by being cheerful.

View life as an exciting challenge rather than as a threat.

Modify your response toward people you find annoying.

Learn how to reprogram your reactions to situations that arise. Find something positive that can come from the situation. Remember that you have a choice in the way you respond. See things from a different perspective; replace negative ideas with positive thoughts. If we think negative thoughts, we will attract negative thought forms; positive thoughts attract positive thought forms that beget the good things and people in our life.

Write affirmations of your own, carry them with you, and read them throughout the day.